The Early Weeks
of Breastfeeding

Excerpt from Working and Breastfeeding Made Simple

Nancy Mohrbacher, IBCLC, FILCA

Praeclarus Press, LLC

www.PraeclarusPress.com

Praeclarus Press, LLC
2504 Sweetgum Lane
Amarillo, Texas 79124 USA
806-367-9950
www.PraeclarusPress.com

DISCLAIMER
The information contained in this publication is advisory only and is not intended to replace sound clinical judgment or individualized patient care. The author disclaims all warranties, whether expressed or implied, including any warranty as the quality, accuracy, safety, or suitability of this information for any particular purpose.

ISBN: 978-1-939807-45-8
©2016 Nancy Mohrbacher. All rights reserved.

Cover Design: Ken Tackett
Acquisition & Development: Kathleen Kendall-Tackett
Copy Editing: Chris Tackett
Layout & Design: Nelly Murariu
Operations: Scott Sherwood

Table of Contents

1

Intro

If you're reading this, chances are you are planning (or have already begun) to breastfeed. Why do you need this book? First, you'll find tips and insights that can simplify your life and make the process less confusing. Second, despite the glut of information available, without some inside knowledge, you're unlikely to meet your breastfeeding goals. I chose this book's content to help you avoid the experience of most women. A 2012 study found that two thirds of American mothers who wanted to exclusively breastfeed for three months didn't (Perrine, Scanlon, Li, Odom, & Grummer-Strawn, 2012).

Employed mothers—especially those working full time—are even less likely to reach their breastfeeding targets than other mothers (Ogbuanu, Glover, Probst, Hussey, & Liu, 2011). In every developed country around the world, breastfeeding rates drop quickly after birth. Even in areas where new mothers receive many months of paid maternity leave, such as the U.K., breastfeeding rates plummet during the early weeks. But before I say more about the challenges and how this book can help you avoid and overcome them, I'd like to share with you the latest on why breastfeeding matters so much to you and your baby.

Why Breastfeeding Matters

Most mothers know that babies who are not breastfed are at greater risk for many health problems. But only recently have we begun to understand the risk to mothers when breastfeeding is cut short. Breastfeeding is not just important to your baby. It's also important to you.

Breastfeeding and You

Breastfeeding is a key women's health issue. A growing body of research has linked a lack of breastfeeding and early weaning to the number one killer of women, heart disease, as well as breast and ovarian cancers, metabolic syndrome, type 2 diabetes, and many other serious health problems. Breastfeeding even affects your response to stress (helping you cope with it better), your resistance to illness (boosting it), and how well and how long you sleep (longer and deeper).

For years, people assumed that breastfeeding was draining to mothers. While fatigue is a normal part of life for all new parents, it turns out this assumption was dead wrong. Your body adapts to lactation by reducing the energy required to make milk, which also improves your other body functions. Scientists think that milk-making actually "primes" or "resets" your metabolism after birth to boost your metabolic efficiency (Stuebe & Rich-Edwards, 2009). Lactation improves digestion and increases absorption of nutrients (Hammond, 1997). It increases your sensitivity to the hormone insulin in the short and long term. For every year you breastfeed, over the next 15 years, your risk of developing type 2 diabetes decreases by about 15% (Stuebe, Rich-Edwards, Willett, Manson, & Michels, 2005).

Breastfeeding and Your Baby

Thousands of studies have reported on the health drawbacks when babies are not breastfed. The American Academy of Pediatrics 2012 Policy Statement recommends exclusive breastfeeding for the first six months and a minimum of one year of total breastfeeding (AAP, 2012). Babies who are *not breastfed* are at increased risk of these health problems.

- 72% increased risk of lower respiratory infections
- 63% increased risk of upper respiratory infections

- 50% increased risk of ear infections
- 40% increased risk of asthma
- 42% increased risk of allergic rashes
- 64% increased risk of digestive tract infections
- 30% increased risk of type 1 diabetes
- 36% increased risk of Sudden Infant Death Syndrome

But a healthier first year is not the end of the story. One compelling reason that one year of breastfeeding is recommended is that these health differences are not restricted to infancy. Babies who do not breastfeed or who wean early are more likely to develop the following conditions as they mature: obesity, diabetes, inflammatory bowel diseases, celiac disease, and childhood leukemia and lymphoma. For an overview of why breastfeeding matters from a health standpoint to both you and your baby, see the 2010 article "The Risks and Benefits of Infant Feeding Practices for Women and Their Children" (Stuebe & Schwarz, 2010): *http://www.ncbi.nlm.nih.gov/pmc/articles/PMC2812877/pdf/RIOG002004_0222.pdf*.

You may find this information disturbing or motivating, but in either case, you need it. In order to make a truly informed decisions, parents need to know how breastfeeding impacts lifelong health. When it comes to breastfeeding, knowledge is definitely power. Knowing what's at stake may help you get through the rough spots that many breastfeeding mothers experience.

For many women, though, the importance of breastfeeding to health isn't even on their radar. Breastfeeding's main appeal is that it increases the connection between mother and baby. When you and your baby are regularly apart, your emotional connection with your baby looms large, as Marge describes.

> I loved that this was something only I could do for my baby. I was worried he would think his nanny was his mom, but everyone reassured me children always know who the mom is—from the intensity of the relationship and connection. Still, the breastfeeding and providing all his milk made me feel connected, a 24/7 mom.
>
> —*Marge G., Ohio, USA*

How can you make breastfeeding—and the close connection that it fosters—a reality? That's what this book is about.

Let Me Be Your Guide

My love for breastfeeding began when I breastfed my own three sons, who are now grown. I started working with mothers as a volunteer in 1982. After I became board-certified, for 10 years, I ran a large private lactation practice in the Chicago area, where I worked one-on-one with thousands of families. I also worked for eight years as a lactation consultant for a major breast pump company, educating health care providers and answering mothers' questions about milk supply and how to make the most of a breast pump. I wrote breastfeeding books used worldwide by parents and professionals, which has kept me current in the lactation research. When I began writing this book, I worked in a corporate lactation program, where I talked daily to women who were pregnant, on maternity leave, and who had returned to work. As you can probably tell, I have a passion for helping breastfeeding mothers. I'd love to share what I've learned with you.

In this book, I've included the key ingredients that make breastfeeding work. It's not complicated. In fact, much of it is very simple. But without this information, working and breastfeeding may be more difficult or more worrisome than it needs to be. These pages include the latest on many of the burning issues you may face: milk production, maternity leave, pumping, flexible job options, childcare, milk storage and handling, work-life balance, and much, much more.

But before we get into these specifics, let me circle back to the sobering figures I mentioned in the beginning on how many women wean earlier than intended. I'd like to explain some of the dynamics that affect these numbers.

The Challenges in Brief

Why is breastfeeding so challenging for so many mothers? One reason is that many mothers and babies don't get the help they need from the institutions that touch their lives. For example, the U.S. Centers for Disease Control and Prevention report that after birth, one in every four U.S. newborns is supplemented in the hospital with infant formula (Centers for Disease Control and Prevention, 2012). Giving newborns formula unnecessarily is a common first step to milk-production problems. Science tells us that worry about milk production is the number one reason women wean before they'd planned. Because many health professionals receive no breastfeeding training, they often give mothers conflicting advice while they are still in the hospital. And some of this advice undermines mothers' best efforts to breastfeed.

After mother and baby arrive home, if breastfeeding problems develop, skilled help is not always affordable or easy to find. When maternity leave ends, many women find their workplaces lack the support they need to continue breastfeeding.

At this writing, a recently upheld U.S. health care law, the Affordable Care Act, is now in place. According to this law, the costs of breastfeeding supplies and services for new mothers should be covered by health insurance. How this law's provisions will translate into reality is still unclear. As always, the devil is in the details.

Weaning earlier than intended, however, is not always the result of health care or worksite challenges. It has a much more personal side. Another major reason so many women stop nursing before they had planned is that they are confused about what's normal and how breastfeeding works (DaMota, Banuelos, Goldbronn, Vera-Beccera, & Heinig, 2012). My hope is that this book will provide an antidote to this confusion so that you can experience the empowerment that comes from reaching your breastfeeding goals.

Maternity Leave

The length of your maternity leave is a big piece of this puzzle. Paid maternity leave is available in almost every country, but the details vary from place to place. In Sweden, for example, one year of paid maternity leave is standard, and fathers also have six months of paid leave. In Canada, depending on how long a mother has been at her job and how many hours per week she works, she may be eligible for 15 weeks of paid leave at full salary with an option to take up to 52 weeks at partial salary and her job guaranteed. Yet not all Canadian mothers take advantage of this.

In the U.K., mothers receive 90% of their weekly salary for the first six weeks after birth and the option of up to 52 weeks maternity leave. After the first six weeks, they can stay home at a flat rate for the next 33 weeks, and the last 13 weeks are unpaid. In Australia, 12 months unpaid leave is guaranteed, and the Australian government pays employers (who pass this on to mothers) up to 18 weeks of pay at the national minimum wage, in addition to whatever job benefits mothers receive. But even where paid maternity leave is available, some women do not take advantage of it.

In the United States, under the Family and Medical Leave Act, 12 weeks of unpaid leave is the law of the land, but that's only for those working full time in companies with more than 50 employees. For many American women, any maternity leave—paid or unpaid—is just a dream. But because maternity leave in the U.S. is tied to job benefits, some have more leeway than others. Women employed at the upper levels of large corporations may receive six months or more of paid leave, while women in low-income jobs may have no leave at all and be forced by money pressures to return to work within weeks—or even days—after giving birth.

How This Book Can Help

My fondest hope is that this book will help you achieve your personal breastfeeding goals. Especially during the early weeks, breastfeeding can sometimes feel like a marathon. But like a marathon, crossing the finish line can be a real peak experience. And like the effort that goes into preparing for a race, the more you put into your breastfeeding relationship, the more you can relish the elation that comes with such an outstanding achievement. Between now and then, I'll be cheering you on.

Nancy Mohrbacher
Arlington Heights, IL USA

2

Birth and
Early Breastfeeding

A fter devoting time to preparing for your birth, what's on your agenda afterwards? Being kind to yourself as you rest and recover is one priority. Being patient as you adjust to motherhood is another. These early postpartum weeks and months may feel like a roller coaster. But this period is key, as it sets the tone for your relationship with your baby, and lays the foundation for long-term breastfeeding. Knowing the basics will help you now and later.

Birth

Does your birth have anything to do with your return to work? It can, especially if you're going back within three months. Melissa M. from New York,

USA returned to work full-time as a claims adjuster for the U.S. Department of Veterans Affairs when her son was 6 weeks and 6 days old. As she put it: "Six weeks to go through the most life and body-changing things was a pittance." At 11 weeks postpartum many women still have childbirth-related symptoms, such as fatigue, headaches, back or neck pain, and abdominal pain (McGovern et al., 2007).

Not surprisingly, after a cesarean section, mothers report more health problems than after a vaginal birth, because they are recovering both from surgery and from having a baby. Today, many more women are having surgical deliveries. The percentages vary widely around the world. The lowest cesarean rate is 14% in the Netherlands and increases from there, with 24% in the U.K., 31% in Australia, 32% in the U.S., and a high of 47% (nearly half!) in Brazil (OECD, 2011). If your baby is born surgically, know that you're far from alone. Be extra kind and patient with yourself, and do everything possible to get extra help while you recover. Double that if your birth was traumatic psychologically, physically, or both.

One way to be kind to yourself is to take it slowly and don't try to jump right back into action. If you'll be returning to work within the first 3 months, take advantage of all offers of help and try to ease back gradually. You might find that your friends and family do not know how they can help, so you may need to ask them to do some specific things for you. Salle Webber's excellent handout, *My Friend is Going to Have a Baby: How Can I Help Her After the Birth?*, can help you get the kind of help you need. Limit visitors to supportive family and friends who will actually pitch in and help rather than expect to be waited on. If your maternity leave is longer than three months, during the first 40 days plan to stay home as much as you can, and if at all possible, arrange for help with household chores and older children. Why 40 days? Read on.

The First 40 Days

In many cultures, the first 40 days after birth are considered a special time distinct from normal life when women are cared for and their housework and childcare responsibilities are assumed by others. Among Latino societies, this time is known as *la cuarentena* (the quarantine). In China, it is known as "doing the month." Even in the U.S., where "overachiever" is our middle name, during the first half of the 20th century it was known as the "lying-in" period. Until recent decades, even American mothers received round-the-clock care and support during the first weeks after giving birth. Postpartum help aids in the physical recovery from childbirth, but the first 40 days are also a time of intense breastfeeding and having help can make the usual feeding frenzies much easier to handle.

To understand what to expect and why breast-feeding is so intense during the early weeks, you need to know how milk production works and how this breastfeeding intensity relates to your supply and your baby's needs. But before discussing milk-making in more depth, let's look at some dynamics unique to this time and how they may affect your priorities.

Timing Is Everything

Do you wonder (like many) if you should devote your maternity leave to getting your baby used to the bottle and establishing the feeding routines you expect later? Many mothers understandably want to do everything possible to make their return to work easier on their baby. Consciously or subconsciously, some even worry about allowing themselves to get too close to their newborn for fear it may be too hard to leave him when the time comes. If you're feeling pressured now to try to prepare yourself and your baby for your separations later, take a deep breath and consider another point of view. This kind of advance preparation may take you in the opposite direction from where you want to go.

Why? Because timing is everything. Different strategies work best at different ages and stages. The amount of milk you produce, your body's responsiveness to breast stimulation, and your baby's needs and adaptability all change over time. What might be a great strategy at 4 months can be a total disaster at 1 week. For that reason, it helps to understand and take full advantage of the unique dynamics of each stage. By planning accordingly, not only will everyone be happier, but it will also be easier to meet your long-term goals. What you do now affects what happens later.

Start by thinking of your maternity leave as a unique bubble of time with your top priority to forge a strong, loving bond with your baby. You have plenty of time later to pump and bottle-feed. (You'll soon read some tips for this.) In fact, almost no one enjoys pumping and bottle-feeding. The time you can focus on just you and your baby is the best part. Don't miss it! Give yourself permission now to get in sync with your newborn. That will strengthen your all-important connection and build a milk supply that will carry you through whatever timeframe you have in mind. By being responsive to your baby's hunger cues, and doing lots of holding and cuddling, you will make the most of this "babymoon." Now on to the nitty-gritty.

How Milk Production Works

During the first 2 weeks after birth, your body is more responsive to breast stimulation than at any other time in your life. The hormones of childbirth prepare your body to produce milk abundantly. In fact, practically speaking, the sky's the limit. Amazingly, by just breastfeeding whenever your baby shows signs of hunger (rooting, hand-to-mouth, fussing), mothers of multiples have produced enough milk for twins, triplets, quadruplets, even quintuplets. During that incredible first two weeks, your body is just waiting for you to tell it how much milk to make. To communicate this, though, you need to know how to speak your body's language.

The Language of Milk Removals

The language your body understands is conveyed through milk removals. The more often and more fully your breasts are drained of milk, the more milk you produce. The less often and less fully the milk is removed, the less milk you produce. Simply put, drained breasts make milk faster, and full breasts make milk slower.

Two aspects of full breasts slow milk production: 1) internal pressure as your breasts fill with milk, and 2) an ingredient in your milk known as feedback inhibitor of lactation, or FIL. As more milk accumulates in your breasts, increasing pressure and FIL send a signal to your breasts to slow milk production. The more pressure and FIL in your breasts, the stronger the signal. The fuller your breasts become, the slower you make milk (Kent, Prime, & Garbin, 2011).

The opposite is also true. Milk production speeds when your milk is removed more often and more fully. When a growing baby starts to need more milk, he feeds more times per day and for longer stretches, taking more of the milk available in your breasts. Table 1 shows how your baby's average milk intake increases during the first 6 months.

Table 1. Baby's average feeding volume by age.

Baby's Age	Average volume per feeding	Average volume per day
1 day	0.2 oz. (10 mL)	2 oz. (50 mL)
3 days	1 oz. (30 mL)	8 oz. (250 mL)
1 week	1.5 oz. (45 mL)	15 oz. (450 mL)
2 weeks	2 oz. (60 mL)	20 oz. (600 mL)
1 month	3-4 oz. (90-120 mL)	25-30 oz. (750-900 mL)
6 months	3-4 oz. (90-120 mL)	30 oz. (900 mL)

Notice that almost all of the increase in milk intake occurs during the first month or so. That's why early breastfeeding is so much more intense then than it will be later. Unlike formula-fed babies, breastfed babies consume about the same amount of milk per day at 1 month as they do at around 6 months (Kent et al., 2013). Yet they continue to grow and thrive, because their rate of growth slows during those months.

How does intense breastfeeding boost your milk production? Usually babies take about two thirds of the milk in the breasts. This means that typically about one third of the milk is left. (Unlike a bottle, your breasts are never empty, so if your baby still seems hungry, put him back to breast again and again.) During the first 40 days, as your baby's appetite increases and his stomach grows, he begins to take more than two thirds of the available milk (maybe three quarters or even nine tenths), which signals your body to make more milk faster. You always produce more than your baby actually needs, and if he takes more of the extra milk, this tells your body to speed milk production.

This natural system, however, only works as it's supposed to if you breastfeed whenever your baby seems hungry rather than on a schedule. At this stage, giving a pacifier regularly can throw this system off, too, because it delays feedings. If the pacifier is given often, this can mean fewer feedings per day, which sends the signal to produce less milk. Giving regular bottles of formula has the same effect. If a baby is not gaining weight well, giving expressed milk or formula can sometimes be necessary. But if your baby is doing well without it, giving formula regularly can undermine your long-term goals by limiting your milk production.

Just to clarify, the first 2 weeks are not the only time you can increase your milk production. It can be done at any stage. Even women who have never been pregnant have produced milk for adopted babies by simply breastfeeding or pumping often. What you need to know is that during the first 2 weeks, bringing your milk production to "full" is easier now than it will ever be again. Your postpartum hormonal levels help get your milk production where you want it for the long term with the least amount of work. Boosting your milk supply takes much less time and effort now than it will later.

There's another reason that it makes sense to make the most of this first 40 days to get to full production quickly. With full production and a more mature baby, breastfeeding becomes much less intense and time consuming. With practice and growth, babies finish feeding in a shorter time. With larger stomachs, they can take more milk and stay content longer with fewer feeds per day. Early breastfeeding can feel overwhelming—something like a marathon—but sticking with it and getting to the "reward period" that starts at around 6 weeks is well worth it. Over the long run, this early investment pays you back many times over in time, cost-savings, and better health for you and your baby.

Breast Storage Capacity

This second major milk-production dynamic is useful to know about now, but is even more important later. The language of milk removals is universal. But feeding patterns among mothers and babies vary a lot, in part because of this physical difference. Understanding breast storage capacity is key to understanding milk production in both the short and long term.

Breast storage capacity is determined by the volume of milk available in your breasts at their fullest time of the day. Storage capacity is not related to breast size, which is determined mostly by how much fatty tissue is in your breasts. Smaller-breasted mothers can have a large storage capacity and larger-breasted mothers can have a small capacity. Storage capacity varies by how much room is in your milk-making glands.

How do differences in storage capacity affect breastfeeding? Not much at first, when your baby's stomach is so small. But after your baby's stomach grows larger, a mother with a large storage capacity will likely notice a very different breastfeeding pattern than a mother with a small storage capacity. Storage capacity may affect feedings in several ways.

- Whether your baby usually takes one breast or both.

- Number of feedings needed each day for your baby to gain weight

- Your baby's longest sleep stretch

Both large-capacity and small-capacity mothers produce plenty of milk. Their babies simply feed differently to get the milk they need. What matters to babies is not how much milk they get per feeding, but how much milk they get in a 24-hour day.

A mother with a large storage capacity has more room in her breasts to hold milk. Because she has more room, in order for there to be enough internal pressure to slow milk production, more milk must accumulate. With so much milk available in her breasts, her baby may always be satisfied with one breast per feeding. He may gain weight well with fewer feedings per day than most babies. And he may sleep for longer stretches at night without her milk production slowing.

The mother with a small storage capacity, on the other hand, will have less milk available at each feeding. For this reason, her baby may want both breasts more often, need more feedings each day to get the same amount of milk, and need to continue night feedings longer. If the baby of the small-capacity mother sleeps for too long, her breasts quickly become so full that milk production slows.

Think of storage capacity as being on a spectrum from very large to very small and every point in between. When you return to work, figuring out where you fall on this spectrum will allow you to customize your daily routine.

Your Baby's Needs and Ability to Adapt

Your baby obviously also plays a major role in how early breastfeeding goes. To understand this better, let's start at the beginning. While in the womb, your baby never felt hunger. He was fed constantly by the nutrients flowing through the umbilical cord. After birth, he feels hunger for the first time. Digesting milk in his stomach and experiencing hunger pangs between feedings are new experiences. To make this transition easier, your breasts start by producing small amounts of milk. Milk production increases over time with frequent nursing.

At birth, small feedings are better for your baby than larger feedings because your newborn's stomach is tiny. An average feeding on the first day of life is about one third of an ounce (10 mL) of colostrum, the early milk you've been making since mid-pregnancy. Colostrum provides concentrated nutrition in amounts perfectly sized to your baby's tiny tummy. With frequent breast-feeding during the first week, your milk production increases every day. As your baby takes more milk per feeding, his stomach gently expands. By his third day, his stomach comfortably holds about an ounce (30 mL) of milk. Your baby's stomach size and your milk production both affect early feeding patterns. Take another look at Table 1 to review the big increase in your milk production during the first month of life.

Attempts to schedule your baby's feedings by the clock during these early weeks are likely to move you further away from your breastfeeding goals. Why? Your baby's stomach is too small to hold enough milk to keep him regularly content for long periods. If feedings are on a schedule, because of your baby's small stomach, he will likely spend some parts of the day hungry and crying, which is stressful for everyone. Also, longer intervals between feedings mean fewer daily milk removals, which will prevent the increases in milk production that are key to meeting your long-term goals. If milk is removed fewer times per day, your body will get the message that you don't need more milk.

After 40 days or so, your baby's stomach will have grown bigger, your milk production will be at its peak, and for many babies a more predictable feeding pattern occurs naturally. Trying to make that happen before its natural time is likely to make life harder for everyone. Also, as your baby matures, he becomes more adaptable to change. Waiting until he's older to make adjustments in his feeding pattern will increase the odds that he can handle them well.

What Breastfeeding Norms Look Like

What should you expect breastfeeding to be like during these first 40 days? When it is going normally, small feedings often mean periods of very frequent and sometimes nonstop nursing. Unlike many babies fed by bottle, most breastfed newborns do not feed at regular time intervals. While it is true that most young babies breastfeed 8 to 12 times every 24 hours, the usual laws of math simply don't apply here.

Cluster Feeding

During the first 40 days or so, your baby probably won't have any sort of regular feeding pattern. This means tracking feedings closely (i.e., number of minutes per breast) provides no real benefit. Most new babies tend to bunch their feedings together at certain times (called cluster nursing), and go longer between feedings at other times. If you're lucky, these longer stretches (up to 4 to 5 hours is fine) will be at night. But don't get your hopes up. At first, because most babies are born with their days and nights mixed up, these longer stretches will probably be during the day.

Your baby wanting to breastfeed soon after a feeding is not a sign that your milk production is low; it's a sign that your baby is doing a good job of bringing in abundant milk.

What's Your Focus?

You'll probably hear all sorts of recommendations about how long to breastfeed, whether to give one or both breasts, or how long is "long enough" to feed on one breast. And how conflicting advice about these sorts of things can be crazy-making, and there are a hundred different baby tracking apps available that record all sorts of information, but give you no context in which to put it.

The truth is that when it comes to early breastfeeding, the clock is not your friend. Why isn't timing important? Because just like grownups, breastfed babies can be fast or slow eaters. Two different babies can consume the same amount of milk in vastly different time frames, from 5 minutes to 45 minutes. It's not helpful to track or even to care how long or how often your baby breastfeeds.

So what *do* you focus on? If this is your first breastfed baby, you may wonder how to know whether breastfeeding is going well. It's good to keep an eye on three things during the first couple of weeks. One is your baby's weight, which is the most reliable way to know how breastfeeding is going. After reaching their low weight on day 3 or 4, breastfed babies gain on average about 1 oz. (30 mL) per day during their first three months. Between weight checks, it's a good idea to keep track of:

- Number of feedings per day (a feeding can mean taking one or both breasts)

- Number of poops

You're looking for a minimum of eight feedings in a 24-hour day. After your baby's poop turns yellow (usually by day 4 or 5), you should expect to see at least three to four poops the size of a U.S. quarter (22 mm) or larger. Your baby's poops are formed from the fatty hindmilk he needs to put on weight. So if you see at least three to four poops per day, you don't need to worry about the number of wet diapers. Because the hindmilk comes after the watery foremilk during feedings, if your baby has the right number of poops, you can assume your baby received plenty of fluids. With both number of feedings and number of poops, you can have too few (and if you do, it's time to arrange for a weight check), but you can't have too many.

Rather than timing breastfeeding by the clock, when all is going well, the recommended feeding strategy is called "finish the first breast first." This means letting your baby breastfeed as long as he likes on the first breast. When he comes off or falls asleep and falls off, offer the other breast. Typically, babies take one breast at some feedings and both breasts at some feedings. By leaving this up to your baby, you can be sure he will get the right amount of milk and will be able to adjust your supply as needed. If your baby is done after one breast, give the other breast at the next feeding. (If baby is clustering feedings together, begin counting the next feeding after at least a 30-minute gap.)

Being back up to birth weight by his 2-week checkup or gaining about an ounce (30 g) per day means your baby is an effective feeder. Once he's proven himself, you don't need to keep track of feedings. Just follow your baby's lead.

Day and Night

What should you expect during the early weeks in terms of feeding patterns? If your baby is typical, feedings will vary by time of day. One of the many differences between breast and bottle is that a breast is not like a faucet, with the milk at the same level day and night. Your milk has its own natural ebb and flow, which affects how your baby's feeds.

During mornings, milk production is usually at its peak. Mothers often report that their babies go longer between feedings in the morning than in the evening, when milk production is at its lowest ebb. Babies get the milk they need in the evening by feeding more often, every hour or even every half hour. This is a completely normal pattern and it does not mean that your milk production is low.

These evening breastfeeding marathons are usually confined to the first 40 days. With growth, your baby's stomach gets bigger and he can hold more milk. And with practice at the breast, your baby learns to get more milk more quickly. With time, your breastfeeding pattern will change, usually becoming more predictable. What's important about this for your baby is not the ebb and flow; it's the total amount of milk he gets every 24 hours.

What About Pumping and Storing?

The early weeks are not the best time to start pumping to store milk. But there are sometimes good reasons to pump now.

Not the Best Time to Store Milk

Why are the first 40 days not the best time to store milk? Review Table 1 again. If your pumping experience is average and you pump between regular feedings, your milk yield will be about half a feeding. If you pump instead of breastfeeding at a usual feeding time, expect to pump a full feeding. At about 1 week, half a feeding is a paltry 0.75 oz. (22.5 mL) of milk. Unless you have a specific reason for providing your baby with extra milk during this time, it is hardly worth the time and effort. (Don't forget, after pumping you still have to clean the pump parts!) Some women who pump early and get average amounts assume wrongly that there's something amiss with their milk production. Even if you know the averages, it's still pretty discouraging. If you wait to start pumping and storing until your milk production increases, you'll get much more milk for your efforts.

What are good reasons to pump? Imagine that your newborn nurses really well from one breast but then is sound asleep and not willing to take the other, very full breast. What do you do? You've basically got two choices. You can express your milk or you can leave your very full breast as is until the next feeding. Allowing your breast to stay overly full for long stretches is not a good plan, because it can lead to a painful condition called mastitis. This is definitely not something you want. Most women experience this as a sore area or lump in one breast, and it can lead to a fever and chills. Any time your breast is full and your baby is not willing to breastfeed, pumping some milk can both keep you comfortable and prevent mastitis from developing, both good things.

One word of caution here. As mentioned, your breasts are much more sensitive to stimulation during the first 2 weeks than they will be at any other time in your life. This means you don't want to overdo it. When mothers do a lot of pumping now, it can lead to oversupply, which means producing much more milk than your baby needs. If you will not be pumping at work and you want to accumulate a huge reserve of milk during maternity leave, lots of pumping now might make sense. If that isn't your situation, there are serious downsides of oversupply for both for you and for your baby. There can definitely be too much of a good thing!

For your baby, a drawback of oversupply is a very fast milk flow. Even without oversupply, it's not uncommon during the first few weeks for babies to sometimes cough, sputter, and pull away from the breast when milk flow becomes overwhelming. But with an oversupply, this can be a constant challenge that leads to unhappiness and breastfeeding struggles.

For you, the drawbacks of oversupply include the possibility that your baby may start clamping down on your nipple during feedings to prevent too-fast milk flow. When you produce much more milk than your baby consumes, this also means that for some parts of the day, your breasts may feel uncomfortably full, which is unpleasant. Staying full for too long can lead to mastitis, described later. To relieve this fullness and prevent mastitis, you may need to pump often, which is another drawback, as pumping is extra work for you and not exactly fun. Depending on how you pump, this may either be part of the problem or part of the solution.

How do you pump to keep yourself comfortable without causing oversupply? It's actually not hard. You use a strategy called "pump to comfort." This means whenever you feel full and your baby is not willing to nurse, you just pump long enough for your breast to feel okay, but not long enough to fully drain it. This might take one minute, three minutes, five minutes, or more. The key is that you stop pumping as soon as you feel comfortable. Draining your breasts fully many times each day can lead to oversupply. Pumping to comfort during the early weeks has no drawbacks other than the work involved. It allows your milk production to adjust to the right level without risk of pain or mastitis, and you can store any milk you pump.

3

FAQ:
Common Early Problems

Hopefully, you won't have the following early breastfeeding challenges, but if you do, here are some fundamentals as a starting point. For more details, you may want to have a basic breastfeeding book on hand, such as *Breastfeeding Made Simple* or *Breastfeeding Solutions*. Another more portable option is the *Breastfeeding Solutions* smartphone app. Links to download it onto Android and iPhones are at: *http://www.nancy mohrbacher.com/app-support* .

Nipple Pain

The most important thing to know about nipple pain is that it is a fixable problem. It's not something you just have to live with.

How much nipple pain is normal during early breastfeeding?

Anything more than mild discomfort during the first minute or two of feedings during the first week or two is a sign that your pain is outside the normal range. Toe-curling pain, pain throughout the feeding, skin trauma or color changes are all signs that it's time to make adjustments. If your own adjustments aren't enough to make breastfeeding comfortable, seek help. Needing breastfeeding help is not a commentary on your mothering skills; a small tweak in how your baby latches is usually all that's needed. Even if someone has already told you that your latch "looks fine," how it looks is not what's important. What matters is how it feels.

What's the connection between baby's latch and sore nipples?

The deeper your nipple extends into your baby's mouth during feedings, the more comfortable breastfeeding should feel. To gauge how deep is deep enough, run your tongue or your finger along the roof of your mouth. The section nearest your front teeth is ridged. Behind these ridges is a smooth area, your hard palate. Closer to your throat, the roof of your mouth becomes soft. The area nicknamed the "comfort zone" is near that part of your baby's mouth where his palate turns from hard to soft. Reaching the comfort zone during breastfeeding protects your nipple from friction and pressure, and your baby gets more milk with each suck.

If your baby latches shallowly, his tongue compresses your nipple against his hard palate, causing nipple distortion and pain. Your nipple may come out of your baby's mouth oddly shaped, smashed looking, or pointed. If your baby breastfeeds with a shallow latch feeding after feeding, this may eventually lead to pain, skin trauma, and bleeding.

How can I get a deeper latch?

Latching a newborn can feel complicated if you're sitting up or lying on your side because gravity pulls your baby down and away from you. Many mothers find that using more relaxed, or laid-back, breastfeeding positions (a term coined by U.K. researcher Suzanne Colson) can make getting a deep latch easier and more automatic during the early weeks. In these positions, gravity works in harmony with your baby's inborn feeding behaviors.

To do this, lean back far enough so your baby's entire weight rests tummy down on your body, but upright enough so that you can see him easily without straining your neck. Think of you and your baby as two puzzle pieces. While experimenting, use these two adjustments to help you find your best fit:

1. **How far you lean back.** Experiment until you find an angle that works for you. Some mothers like their head and shoulders higher or lower.

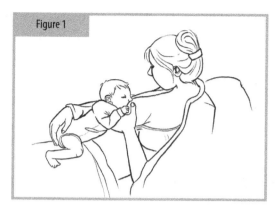

Figure 1

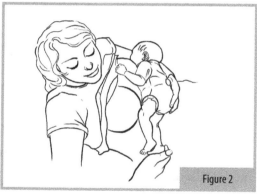

Figure 2

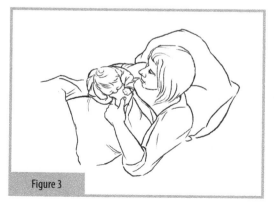

Figure 3

2. **From which direction your baby approaches the breast.** Put your baby lengthwise, diagonally, or across your torso until you find a position he likes (Figures 1, 2, & 3).

When you lay your baby tummy down near your exposed breasts, your baby's inborn feeding behaviors are triggered and he may bob his way to the breast. If he seems to need your help, feel free to give it. Nature hardwires babies to get to the breast and feed in these more natural positions. When your baby's feeding behaviors are triggered and he has an active role in taking the breast, many mothers find they achieve an even deeper latch than when they try to micromanage it while in a sitting-straight-up position.

You'll know you have a deeper latch when breastfeeding feels more comfortable than before. If you have nipple trauma, breastfeeding may not yet feel completely comfortable. Any reduction in pain indicates you've reached the comfort zone. By getting your nipple into the comfort zone at every breastfeeding, your nipples can heal even while continuing to breastfeed.

Are there other causes of nipple pain?

Yes. One easy-to-correct cause is not breaking your baby's suction first when you take your baby off the breast. Another is having your pump suction up too high or using a pump with a too-small nipple tunnel. Overzealous cleaning of your nipples or the use harsh products can also cause soreness. Another cause is lack of blood flow to the nipple, which can be due to circulatory problems. (If this is the cause, when the pain starts, your nipple will turn white, blue, or red.) Some babies are tongue-tied, which can also cause nipple soreness, even with a deep latch. A lactation consultant should be able to check your baby for this anatomical variation. You can read more about tongue tie in this online article: _https://breastfeedingusa.org/ content/article/tell-me-about-tongue-ties._ Other causes of pain include infected nipples or a clogged nipple pore (white spot on the nipple).

What should I do if I can't get comfortable?

If you have tried getting a deeper latch on your own and you're still in pain, it's time to seek skilled breastfeeding help. You can find a board-certified lactation consultant in your area by going to the website, _www.ilca.org,_ click on its "Find a Lactation Consultant" page, and enter your ZIP or postal code.

Some products, such as ultrapurified lanolin and hydrogel pads, can be soothing when you're sore, but unless you correct the cause of the problem, they will only help temporarily.

Engorgement

Engorgement is not an inevitable part of early breast-feeding. Severe engorgement usually only happens when your baby does not breastfeed often or effectively in the early days.

How will I know if I have engorgement?

When it happens, engorgement usually starts around the third or fourth day after birth. Most mothers feel breast fullness around this time, but if your breasts are very full, very firm, painful, hard, or hot, you may be engorged. Engorgement is not just caused by an increase in your milk production. Other body fluids, such as extra blood and lymph, are also drawn to your breasts as your milk production ramps up, contributing to congestion there.

Engorgement can make the area around your nipple (areola) firm, making a deep latch difficult, and sometimes causing the nipple to flatten. To get a deep latch, the areola must be soft enough to change shape during suckling, so the nipple can extend into the "comfort zone."

What's the best way to treat engorgement?

When engorged, many mothers worry about breast-feeding more often and expressing milk, because they're concerned they may make it worse. But the best thing you can do to relieve engorgement is to drain your breasts often and well. Try these treatments.

- **Breastfeed your baby at least 8 to 12 times a day** (more is better), every 1.5 to 2 hours during the day and 2 to 3 hours at night until you feel relief. Make sure your baby has a deep latch.

- **If a deep latch is difficult, use reverse pressure softening** to move the swelling away from your nipples. This simple technique was developed by K. Jean Cotterman, RNC, IBCLC. You can see a video demonstration at: _http://on.aol.com/video/ how-to-use-reverse-pressure-softening-during-en gorgement-106182017_

- **If your baby is not breastfeeding well or at all, use an effective breast pump** to drain your breasts well at least eight times per day.

- **Avoid bottles, pacifiers, or formula supplements** to keep your baby at the breast.

- **Apply warmth before feedings to aid milk flow and cool between feedings to reduce swelling.**

- **Take an anti-inflammatory medication**, such as ibuprofen. Ask your health care provider to recommend one.

- **Wear a supportive bra** that fits you well and is not too tight.

If you follow the above suggestions, your symptoms should begin to clear within a day or two. If they don't, contact a breastfeeding specialist.

Mastitis

About one in five breastfeeding mothers develops mastitis at some point, so if you develop this condition, know that you're not alone.

What is mastitis?

Mastitis refers to an inflammation of the breast, with or without a fever. A mild form of mastitis—a tender spot or lump in your breast with no fever—is sometimes referred to as a plugged, clogged, or blocked duct. If you have a temperature of more than 101°F (38.4°C), are achy, or have other symptoms that feel like the flu, you probably have a more severe case that has progressed into an infection. Other signs of infection include a cracked nipple with pus, pus or blood in your milk, red streaks on your breast, and severe symptoms that appear suddenly.

How can I treat mastitis?

For mastitis with and without infection, the treatment is generally the same. However, if you think you have an infection, call your health care provider and ask about a prescription of antibiotics, and then follow the suggestions below.

- **Breastfeed frequently on the affected breast**. Drain that breast often by breastfeeding or pumping. Letting milk accumulate in your breast will make it worse. If breastfeeding is uncomfortable, use whichever positions are most comfortable. If your baby refuses to nurse on your affected side, pump until the infection heals.

- **Ask your health care provider about using a pain reliever, such as ibuprofen.**

- **Apply heat to the area and gently massage it** from your armpit to your nipple. Use warm compresses at least 3 times a day.

- **Breastfeed your baby right after the heat treatment** to help loosen the plug.

- **Wear loose clothing.** Consider whether your bra might be too tight, which is one possible cause of mastitis.

- **Rest.** This enhances your body's natural defenses.

What causes mastitis?

One key to avoiding mastitis in the future is to determine why you got it in the first place. These are the most common causes.

- Nipple trauma, which lets organisms enter the breast

- Consistent pressure on your breast for long periods, such as from a bra that's too tight, a strap that cuts across your chest, or sleeping on your stomach

- Prolonged breast fullness from irregular feeding patterns or suddenly going longer between feedings (your baby sleeping through the night, busy holidays, the use of supplements or a pacifier). If you can determine the cause, you may be able to prevent mastitis from occurring again.

See the Resources section for how to find skilled breastfeeding help in your area when needed.

4

How to Hand Express Milk

Hand expression can be a useful way to relieve breast fullness, boost milk production, and provide milk for your baby. Here's how to do it.

Getting ready

First, wash your hands well. Find a clean collection container with a wide mouth, like a cup. If possible, express in a private, comfortable place where you can relax. Feeling relaxed enhances milk flow.

Find your sweet spot

Whichever hand-expression technique you use, the key is finding your "sweet spot," the area on your breast where milk flows fastest when it is compressed. Try different finger positions until you find it. If the dark area around your nipple (areola) is large, your sweet spot may be inside it. If it is small, your sweet spot may be outside it.

Do what works best and expresses the most milk

This method combines the World Health Organization technique with others:

1. Before expressing, gently massage your breasts with your hands and fingertips or a soft baby brush or warm towel.

2. Sit up and lean slightly forward, so gravity helps milk flow.

3. To find your sweet spot, start with your thumb on top of the breast and fingers below, both about 1.5 inches (4 cm) from the base of the nipple. Some mothers find it helpful to curl their hand and use just the tips of their fingers and thumb. Apply steady pressure several times into the breast toward the chest wall. If no milk comes, shift finger and thumb either closer to or farther from the nipple and compress

again a few times. Repeat, moving finger and thumb until you feel slightly firmer breast tissue and gentle pressure yields milk. After finding your sweet spot, skip the "finding" phase and start with your fingers on this area.

4. Apply steady pressure on areas of milk in the breast by pressing fingers toward the chest wall, not toward the nipple.

5. While applying inward pressure on the breast, compress thumb and finger pads together (pushing in, not pulling out toward the nipple). Find a good rhythm of press—compress—relax, like a baby's suckling rhythm.

6. Switch breasts every few minutes (5 or 6 times in total at each expression) while rotating finger position around the breast. After expressing, all areas of the breast should feel soft. This process usually takes about 20 to 30 minutes.

If needed, adjust

Hand expression should feel comfortable. If not, you may be compressing too hard, sliding your fingers along the skin, or squeezing the nipple. If you feel discomfort, review the instructions, and adjust your technique. It is important to find the method that works best for you. You can find several demonstration videos online by doing a search for "hand expression of breast milk."

5

Resources

Finding Skilled Breastfeeding Help

If you're in need of breastfeeding help, don't wait to find someone. Usually, the sooner you get help, the easier it is to solve your problem. When contacting local breastfeeding specialists, be aware that different credentials reflect different levels of education and training. A variety of initials (CLC, CLE, CBE, CBC, LE, and others) are awarded after attending a brief training course, usually less than one week long. A person with these initials may be able to provide some help but may have limited skills, understanding, and experience.

The credential IBCLC, however, indicates—at the least—a basic competence in the field of lactation. These initials stand for "International Board Certified Lactation Consultant." To receive this credential, a person must pass an all-day certifying exam. To qualify to take that exam, she must first have a combination of formal education, breastfeeding education, and thousands of hours working one-on-one with breastfeeding mothers and babies. There are several ways you can find a local IBCLC.

- Click on the "Find a Lactation Consultant" link on *www.ilca.org* and enter your ZIP or postal code. ILCA is the International Lactation Consultant Association, the professional association for lactation consultants. Not all international board certified lactation consultants are members.

- Contact your local birthing facility and ask to speak to the breastfeeding specialist. Ask if she can help you or if she knows someone in your community who can.

- Contact your local public-health department and ask if there is any IBCLCs on staff who can help you.

- Contact mother-to-mother breastfeeding support people in your area (see next section) and ask them for suggestions. They may know the best choices in your area.

Another possible source of skilled breastfeeding help is the mother-to-mother support organizations listed in the next section. These experienced breastfeeding mothers work as volunteers to help other mothers. Their skill level can run the gamut from highly skilled to inexperienced. Hopefully, if they can't help you, they'll know someone who can.

Getting the Support You Need

Don't underestimate the importance of ongoing breastfeeding support. What's really great today is that breastfeeding support comes in many forms. Even if you are in a remote location, work odd hours, or lack safe, reliable transportation, you can access the many Facebook groups and online forums that support employed breastfeeding mothers. To get a sense of what's out there and its immense value, see Lara Audelo's book, *The Virtual Breastfeeding Culture: Seeking Mother-to-Mother Support in the Digital Age.*

Mother-to-Mother Breastfeeding Organizations

It's always a plus to have choices, and sometimes there's just no substitute for spending face time with other mothers and babies. Mother-to-mother breast-feeding organizations that offer in-person meetings (as well as online and Facebook support options) are:

- Breastfeeding USA (*www.breastfeedingusa.org*), this rapidly growing nonprofit organization was formed in 2010 with a focus on providing evidence-based information and support in a variety of formats.

- Australian Breastfeeding Association (_www.breastfeeding.asn.au_). This long-standing beacon of breastfeeding support offers a range of services, such as classes, email counseling, a 24-hour Breastfeeding Helpline, online forums, and local support groups.

In the U.K., there are several national breastfeeding support organizations. A list of their links is at: _http://www.nhs.uk/Conditions/pregnancy-and-baby/pages/breastfeeding-help-support.aspx#close_

Another mother-to-mother option in most countries is La Leche League International (_www.llli.org_), the grandmother of breastfeeding support, which has been helping mothers since 1956 and offers in-person meetings, phone, and email help. One way La Leche League differs from other breastfeeding organizations is that it requires its leaders to follow its parenting philosophy, which is consistent with attachment parenting. It does not require those who seek help from La Leche League to follow its philosophy.

Doulas

"Doula" comes from the Greek word for servant, and refers to someone who provides practical and emotional help to women before, during, and after birth. Many doulas also offer breastfeeding help and support.

- DONA International (*www.dona.org*) lists labor-support and postpartum doulas.

- Find a Doula, Australia (*http://www.findadoula.com.au/*) to locale doulas in Australia.

- Doula U.K. (*http://doula.org.uk/*) to locate labor and postpartum/postnatal doulas.

Websites

The internet can be an unreliable place. All breast-feeding websites are definitely not created equal! Here are some that you can trust.

- *Kellymom.com* is a great site that includes articles on almost every aspect of breastfeeding.

- *NancyMohrbacher.com* includes a section for employed breastfeeding mothers and many articles on hot topics.

- *BreastfeedingMadeSimple.com* is the companion site for the book I co-authored with Kathleen Kendall-Tackett, *Breastfeeding Made Simple*. It has many resources for a wide range of breastfeeding concerns and common challenges.

- *WomensHealth.gov/breastfeeding/government-in-action/business-case.html* Here you can download *The Business Case for Breastfeeding*, which includes materials for mothers, human resources, CEOs, etc. A treasure trove of great resources.

- *Womenshealth.gov/breastfeeding/employer-solutions/index.php* A new U.S. Government website for working and breastfeeding mothers and their employers.

- *BestforBabes.org* offers resources for employed mothers, as well as ways to avoid "booby traps."

- *BreastfeedingPartners.org* Click on the "Work & School" tab to find its *Making It Work Toolkit,* a great resource.

- *Workandpump.com* This site is an oldie but a goodie that is chock full of great info.

- *BreastfeedingUSA.org* offers many helpful articles and a locator for local support.

- *Breastfeedinginc.ca* has many helpful articles and videos by Canadian pediatrician and lactation consultant, Dr. Jack Newman.

- *Isisonline.org.uk* offers evidence-based information for parents and professionals about infant sleep norms.

- *Lowmilksupply.org* was created by two lactation consultants who specialize in milk production issues.

Free Online Videos

Hand Expression:

http://newborns.stanford.edu/Breastfeeding/HandExpression.html

Hands-on Pumping:

http://newborns.stanford.edu/Breastfeeding/MaxProduction.html

Paced Bottle Feeding for the Breastfed Baby:

http://www.youtube.com/watch?v=UH4T70OSzGs&feature=youtube

Reverse Pressure Softening. How to Relieve Engorgement:

*http://www.youtube.com/watch?v=2_*
RD9HNrOJ8&oref=http%3A%2F%2Fwww.youtube.
com%2Fwatch%3Fv%3D2_RD9HNrOJ8&has_verified=1

Books

These resources would be great additions to any employed mother's bookshelf.

Audelo, L. (2013). *The virtual breastfeeding culture: Seeking mother-to-mother support in the digital age.* Amarillo, TX Praeclarus Press.

Mohrbacher, N., & Kendall-Tackett, K. (2010). *Breastfeeding made simple: Seven natural laws for nursing mothers, 2nd Ed.* Oakland, CA: New Harbinger Publications.

Mohrbacher, N. (2013). *Breastfeeding solutions: Quick tips for the most common nursing challenges.* Oakland, CA: New Harbinger Publications.

Peterson, A., & Harmer, M. (2010). *Balancing breast and bottle: Reaching your breastfeeding goals.* Amarillo, TX: Hale Publishing.

Rapley, G., & Murkett, T. (2010). *Baby-led weaning: The essential guide to introducing solid foods—and helping your baby to grow up a happy and confident eater.* New York: The Experiment.

Roche-Paull, R. (2010). *Breastfeeding in combat boots: A survival guide to successful breastfeeding while serving in the military.* Amarillo, TX: Hale Publishing.

West, D., & Marasco, L. (2009). *The breastfeeding mothers' guide to making more milk.* New York: McGraw-Hill.

Smartphone App

Here's a basic breastfeeding resource you can download to your Android or iPhone. It covers the 30 most common breastfeeding challenges, and includes the milk-storage guidelines. Use your smartphone to open this link and you're on your way.

Breastfeeding Solutions by Nancy Mohrbacher. (2013). Available for Android and iPhones from Amazon, Google Play, and the App Store. *http://www.nancymohrbacher.com/app-support/*

Breast Pumps to Buy or Rent

Here is the contact information for the three recommended breast-pump brands.

Ameda Breast Pumps

To locate an Ameda rental pump or purchase an Ameda Purely Yours pump near you, call Ameda Breastfeeding Products, at 1-866-99AMEDA (1-866-992-6332), or go online to _www.Ameda.com_.

Hygeia Breast Pumps

To locate a Hygeia rental pump or a Hygeia Enjoye purchase pump near you, call Hygeia at 1-888-786-7466 or go online to _www.Hygeiainc.com_.

Medela Breast Pumps

To locate a Medela rental pump or purchase a Medela Pump In Style or Freestyle pump near you, contact Medela, Inc., at 1-800-TELLYOU (in the U.S.) or go online to _www.medela.com_.

Other Products

Hands-Free Pumping Devices

For the latest commercial products that help you pump hands-free, just Google "hands-free pumping." Some women make their own. Here are two options:

- This free tutorial uses elastic hair bands: *http:// kellymom.com/bf/pumpingmoms/pumping/hands-free-pumping/*

- This one (be sure to click on the pictures) uses rubber bands: *http://www.workandpump.com/handsfree.htm*

Prevent Milk Leakage

To find LilyPadz, the silicone product that applies pressure to the nipples to prevent milk leakage, go online to *www.lilypadz.com*.

Collect Leaked Milk

To find Milkies milk savers, the container you wear to collect milk while your baby breastfeeds, go online to *http://www.mymilkies.com/milksaver*.

References

American Academy of Pediatrics (AAP). (2012). Breastfeeding and the use of human milk. *Pediatrics, 129*(3), e827-e841.

American Academy of Pediatrics. (AAP). (2011). SIDS and other sleep-related infant deaths: expansion of recommendations for a safe infant sleeping environment. *Pediatrics, 128*(5), 1030-1039.

American Academy of Pediatrics. (AAP). (2001). The use and misuse of fruit juice in pediatrics. *Pediatrics, 107*(5), 1210-1213.

Blyton, D. M., Sullivan, C. E., & Edwards, N. (2002). Lactation is associated with an increase in slow-wave sleep in women. *Journal of Sleep Research, 11*(4), 297-303.

Boushey, H., & Glynn, S. J. (2012). There are significant business costs to replacing employees. Retrieved from: http://www.americanprogress.org/wp-content/uploads/2012/11/CostofTurnover.pdf

Brusseau, R. (1998). *Bacterial analysis of refrigerated human milk following infant feeding. Unpublished senior thesis.* Concordia University.

Centers for Disease Control and Prevention. (CDC). (2013). *Unmarried childbearing.* Retrieved from: http://www.cdc.gov/nchs/fastats/unmarry.htm

Centers for Disease Control and Prevention. (CDC). (2012). *Percentage of breastfed U.S. children who are supplemented with infant formula, by birth year.* Retrieved from http://www.cdc.gov/breastfeeding/data/nis_data/

Chatterji, P., & Markowitz, S. (2012). Family leave after childbirth and the mental health of new mothers. *The Journal of Mental Health Policy and Economics, 15*(2), 61-76.

Cohen, R., Lange, L., & Slusser, W. (2002). A description of a male-focused breastfeeding promotion corporate lactation program. *Journal of Human Lactation, 18*(1), 61-65.

Cohen, R., & Mrtek, M. B. (1994). The impact of two corporate lactation programs on the incidence and duration of breast-feeding by employed mothers. *American Journal of Health Promotion, 8*(6), 436-441.

Cohen, R., Mrtek, M. B., & Mrtek, R. G. (1995). Comparison of maternal absenteeism and infant illness rates among breast-feeding and formula-feeding women in two corporations. *American Journal of Health Promotion, 10*(2), 148-153.

Colson, S. D., Meek, J. H., & Hawdon, J. M. (2008). Optimal positions for the release of primitive neonatal reflexes stimulating breastfeeding. *Early Human Development, 84*(7), 441-449.

DaMota, K., Banuelos, J., Goldbronn, J., Vera-Beccera, L. E., & Heinig, M. J. (2012). Maternal request for in-hospital supplementation of healthy breastfed infants among low-income women. *Journal of Human Lactation, 28*(4), 476-482.

Dewey, K. G., & Brown, K. H. (2003). Update on technical issues concerning complementary feeding of young children in developing countries and implications for intervention programs. *Food and Nutrition Bulletin, 24*(1), 5-28.

Doan, T., Gardiner, A., Gay, C. L., & Lee, K. A. (2007). Breast-feeding increases sleep duration of new parents. *Journal of Perinatal and Neonatal Nursing, 21*(3), 200-206.

Dunn, B. F., Zavela, K. J., Cline, A. D., & Cost, P. A. (2004). Breastfeeding practices in Colorado businesses. *Journal of Human Lactation, 20*(2), 170-177.

Geddes, D. T. (2009). The use of ultrasound to identify milk ejection in women: Tips and pitfalls. *International Breastfeeding Journal, 4*, 5.

Goldblum, R. M., Garza, C., Johnson, C. A., Harrist, R., & Nichols, B. L. (1981). Human milk banking I: Effects of container upon immunologic factors in mature milk. *Nutrition Research, 1*, 449-459.

Hale, T. W. (2012). *Medications & Mothers' Milk* (15th Ed.). Amarillo, TX: Hale Publishing.

Hammond, K. A. (1997). Adaptation of the maternal intestine during lactation. *Journal of Mammary Gland Biology and Neoplasia, 2*(3), 243-252.

Heinig, M. J., Nommsen, L. A., Peerson, J. M., Lonnerdal, B., & Dewey, K. G. (1993). Energy and protein intakes of breast-fed and formula-fed infants during the first year of life and their association with growth velocity: the DARLING Study. *American Journal of Clinical Nutrition, 58*(2), 152-161.

Hennart, P., Delogne-Desnoeck, J., Vis, H., & Robyn, C. (1981). Serum levels of prolactin and milk production in women during a lactation period of thirty months. *Clinical Endocrinology (Oxf), 14*(4), 349-353.

Hicks, J. B. (Ed.). (2006). *Hirikani's daughters: Women who scale modern mountains to combine breastfeeding and working.* Schaumburg, Illinois: La Leche League International.

Hill, P. D., Aldag, J. C., Chatterton, R. T., & Zinaman, M. (2005). Comparison of milk output between mothers of preterm and term infants: The first 6 weeks after birth. *Journal of Human Lactation, 21*(1), 22-30.

HRSA. (2008). *The Business Case for Breastfeeding.* Retrieved from: http://www.womenshealth.gov/breastfeeding/government-in-action/business-case-for-breastfeeding/.

Islam, M. M., Peerson, J. M., Ahmed, T., Dewey, K. G., & Brown, K. H. (2006). Effects of varied energy density of complementary foods on breast-milk intakes and total energy consumption by healthy, breastfed Bangladeshi children. *American Journal of Clinical Nutrition, 83*(4), 851-858.

Jones, E., & Hilton, S. (2009). Correctly fitting breast shields are the key to lactation success for pump dependent mothers following preterm delivery. *Journal of Neonatal Nursing, 15*(1), 14-17.

Jones, F., & Tully, M. R. (2011). *Best practices for expressing, storing and handling human milk* (3rd Ed.). Raleigh, NC: Human Milk Banking Association of North America.

Kearney, M. H., & Cronenwett, L. (1991). Breastfeeding and employment. *Journal of Obstetric, Gynecologic & Neonatal Nursing, 20*(6), 471-480.

Kendall-Tackett, K., Cong, Z., & Hale, T. W. (2011). The effect of feeding method on sleep duration, maternal well-being, and postpartum depression. *Clinical Lactation, 2*(2), 22-26.

Kent, J. C. (2007). How breastfeeding works. *Journal of Midwifery & Women's Health, 52*(6), 564-570.

Kent, J. C., Hepworth, A. R., Sherriff, J. L., Cox, D. B., Mitoulas, L. R., & Hartmann, P. E. (2013). Longitudinal changes in breastfeeding patterns from 1 to 6 months of lactation. *Breastfeeding Medicine, 8,* 401-407.

Kent, J. C., Mitoulas, L., Cox, D. B., Owens, R. A., & Hartmann, P. E. (1999). Breast volume and milk production during extended lactation in women. *Experimental Physiology, 84*(2), 435-447.

Kent, J. C., Mitoulas, L. R., Cregan, M. D., Geddes, D. T., Larsson, M., Doherty, D. A., et al. (2008). Importance of vacuum for breast milk expression. *Breastfeeding Medicine, 3*(1), 11-19.

Kent, J. C., Mitoulas, L. R., Cregan, M. D., Ramsay, D. T., Doherty, D. A., & Hartmann, P. E. (2006). Volume and frequency of breastfeedings and fat content of breast milk throughout the day. *Pediatrics, 117*(3), e387-395.

Kent, J. C., Prime, D. K., & Garbin, C. P. (2011). Principles for maintaining or increasing breast milk production. *Journal of Obstetric, Gynecologic, & Neonatal Nursing.* doi: 10.1111/j.1552-6909.2011.01313.x.

Kent, J. C., Ramsay, D. T., Doherty, D., Larsson, M., & Hartmann, P. E. (2003). Response of breasts to different stimulation patterns of an electric breast pump. *Journal of Human Lactation, 19*(2), 179-186.

Kimbro, R. T. (2006). On-the-job moms: Work and breastfeeding initiation and duration for a sample of low-income women. *Maternal & Child Health Journal, 10*(1), 19-26.

Kline, T. S., & Lash, S. R. (1964). The bleeding nipple of pregnancy and postpartum period: A cytologic and histologic study. *Acta Cytologica, 8,* 336-340.

Kramer, M. S., Guo, T., Platt, R. W., Vanilovich, I., Sevkovskaya, Z., Dzikovich, I., et al. (2004). Feeding effects on growth during infancy. *Journal of Pediatrics, 145*(5), 600-605.

Kramer, M. S., & Kakuma, R. (2012). Optimal duration of exclusive breastfeeding *Cochrane Database of Systematic Reviews, Art No. CD003517.*

La Leche League International. (LLLI). (2008). *Storing human milk.* Schaumburg, IL: Author.

Lawrence, R. A., & Lawrence, R. M. (2011). *Breastfeeding: A guide for the medical profession* (7th Ed.). Philadelphia, PA: Elsevier Mosby.

Li, R., Fein, S. B., & Grummer-Strawn, L. M. (2008). Association of breastfeeding intensity and bottle-emptying behaviors at early infancy with infants' risk for excess weight at late infancy. *Pediatrics, 122 Suppl 2,* S77-84.

Li, R., Magadia, J., Fein, S. B., & Grummer-Strawn, L. M. (2012). Risk of bottle-feeding for rapid weight gain during the first year of life. *Archives of Pediatric & Adolescent Medicine, 166*(5), 431-436.

Macknin, M. L., Medendorp, S. V., & Maier, M. C. (1989). Infant sleep and bedtime cereal. *American Journal of Diseases of Children, 143*(9), 1066-1068.

Manohar, A. A., Williamson, M., & Koppikar, G. V. (1997). Effect of storage of colostrum in various containers. *Indian Pediatrics, 34*(4), 293-295.

McGovern, P., Dowd, B., Gjerdingen, D., Dagher, R., Ukestad, L., McCaffrey, D., et al. (2007). Mothers' health and work-related factors at 11 weeks postpartum. *The Annals of Family Medicine, 5*(6), 519-527.

McGovern, P., Dowd, B., Gjerdingen, D., Gross, C. R., Kenney, S., Ukestad, L., et al. (2006). Postpartum health of employed mothers 5 weeks after childbirth. *Annals of Family Medicine, 4*(2), 159-167.

McGovern, P., Dowd, B., Gjerdingen, D., Dagher, R., Ukestad, L., McCaffrey, D., et al. (2007). Mothers' health and work-related factors at 11 weeks postpartum. *Annals of Family Medicine, 5*(6), 519-527.

McKenna, J. J., & McDade, T. (2005). Why babies should never sleep alone: A review of the co-sleeping controversy in relation to SIDS, bedsharing and breast feeding. *Paediatric Respiratory Reviews, 6*(2), 134-152.

Meier, P. (1988). Bottle- and breast-feeding: Effects on transcutaneous oxygen pressure and temperature in preterm infants. *Nursing Research, 37*(1), 36-41.

Meier, P., & Anderson, G. C. (1987). Responses of small preterm infants to bottle- and breast-feeding. *MCN American Journal of Maternal Child Nursing, 12*(2), 97-105.

Meier, P., Motykowski, J. E., & Zuleger, J. L. (2004). Choosing a correctly-fitted breast shield for milk expression. *Medela Messenger, 21,* 8-9.

Mohrbacher, N. (2011). The magic number and long-term milk production. *Clinical Lactation, 2*(1), 15-18.

Mohrbacher, N. (2010). *Breastfeeding answers made simple.* Amarillo, TX: Hale Publishing.

Molbak, K., Gottschau, A., Aaby, P., Hojlyng, N., Ingholt, L., & da Silva, A. P. (1994). Prolonged breast feeding, diarrhoeal disease, and survival of children in Guinea-Bissau. *British Medical Journal, 308*(6941), 1403-1406.

Morton, J., Hall, J. Y., Wong, R. J., Thairu, L., Benitz, W. E., & Rhine, W. D. (2009). Combining hand techniques with electric pumping increases milk production in mothers of preterm infants. *Journal of Perinatology, 29*(11), 757-764.

Morton, J., Wong, R. J., Hall, J. Y., Pang, W. W., Lai, C. T., Lui, J., et al. (2012). Combining hand techniques with electric pumping increases the caloric content of milk in mothers of preterm infants. *Journal of Perinatology, 32*(10), 791-796.

Neville, M. C., Allen, J. C., Archer, P. C., Casey, C. E., Seacat, J., Keller, R. P., et al. (1991). Studies in human lactation: milk volume and nutrient composition during weaning and lactogenesis. *American Journal of Clinical Nutrition, 54*(1), 81-92.

Nichols, M. R., & Roux, G. M. (2004). Maternal perspectives on postpartum return to the workplace. *Journal of Obstetric, Gynecologic, & Neonatal Nursing, 33*(4), 463-471.

Nielsen, S. B., Reilly, J. J., Fewtrell, M. S., Eaton, S., Grinham, J., & Wells, J. C. (2011). Adequacy of milk intake during exclusive breastfeeding: A longitudinal study. *Pediatrics, 128*(4), e907-914.

NWLC. (2012). *The next generation of Title IX: Pregnant and parenting students* [Electronic Version].Retrieved from: http://www.titleix.info/history/history-overview.aspx

Odom, E. C., Li, R., Scanlon, K. S., Perrine, C. G., & Grummer-Strawn, L. (2013). Reasons for earlier than desired cessation of breastfeeding. *Pediatrics, 131*(3), e726-732.

OECD. (2011). *Health at a glance 2011: OECD Indicators: 4.9 Caesarean sections.* Retrieved from: http://www.oecd-ilibrary. org/sites/health_glance-2011-en/04/09/g4-09-01.html?itemId=/content/chapter/health_glance-2011-37-en

Ogbuanu, C., Glover, S., Probst, J., Liu, J., & Hussey, J. (2011). The effect of maternity leave length and time of return to work on breastfeeding. *Pediatrics, 127*(6), e1414-1427.

Ogbuanu, C., Glover, S., Probst, J., Hussey, J., & Liu, J. (2011). Balancing work and family: Effect of employment characteristics on breastfeeding. *Journal of Human Lactation, 27*(3), 225-238; quiz 293-225.

Ortiz, J., McGilligan, K., & Kelly, P. (2004). Duration of breast milk expression among working mothers enrolled in an employer-sponsored lactation program. *Pediatric Nursing, 30*(2), 111-119.

PAHO/WHO. (2001). *Guiding principles for complementary feeding of the breastfed child.* Retrieved from: http://whqlibdoc.who. int/paho/2004/a85622.pdf.

Paxson, C. L., Jr., & Cress, C. C. (1979). Survival of human milk leukocytes. *Journal of Pediatrics, 94*(1), 61-64.

Perrine, C. G., Scanlon, K. S., Li, R., Odom, E., & Grummer-Strawn, L. M. (2012). Baby-Friendly hospital practices and meeting exclusive breastfeeding intention. *Pediatrics, 130*(1), 54-60.

Peterson, A., & Harmer, M. (2010). *Balancing breast & bottle: Reaching your breastfeeding goals.* Amarillo, TX: Hale Publishing.

Pittard, W. B., 3rd, & Bill, K. (1981). Human milk banking. Effect of refrigeration on cellular components. *Clinical Pediatrics, 20*(1), 31-33.

Prime, D. K., Kent, J. C., Hepworth, A. R., Trengove, N. J., & Hartmann, P. E. (2012). Dynamics of milk removal during simultaneous breast expression in women. *Breastfeeding Medicine, 7*(2), 100-106.

Quan, R., Yang, C., Rubinstein, S., Lewiston, N. J., Sunshine, P., Stevenson, D. K., et al. (1992). Effects of microwave radiation on anti-infective factors in human milk. *Pediatrics, 89*(4 Pt 1), 667-669.

Rechtman, D. J., Lee, M. L., & Berg, H. (2006). Effect of environmental conditions on unpasteurized donor human milk. *Breastfeeding Medicine, 1*(1), 24-26.

Roe, B., Whittington, L. A., Fein, S. B., & Teisl, M. F. (1999). Is there competition between breast-feeding and maternal employment? *Demography, 36*(2), 157-171.

SHRM. (2013). *2012 employee benefits research report.* Retrieved from: http://www.shrm.org/research/surveyfindings/articles/pages/2012employeebenefitsresearchreport.aspx

Sievers, E., Oldigs, H. D., Santer, R., & Schaub, J. (2002). Feeding patterns in breast-fed and formula-fed infants. *Annals of Nutrition and Metabolism, 46*(6), 243-248.

Skafida, V. (2012). Juggling work and motherhood: The impact of employment and maternity leave on breastfeeding duration: A survival analysis on Growing Up in Scotland data. *Maternal and Child Health Journal, 16*(2), 519-527.

Slusser, W. M., Lange, L., Dickson, V., Hawkes, C., & Cohen, R. (2004). Breast milk expression in the workplace: A look at frequency and time. *Journal of Human Lactation, 20*(2), 164-169.

Stuebe, A. M., & Rich-Edwards, J. W. (2009). The reset hypothesis: Lactation and maternal metabolism. *American Journal of Perinatology, 26*(1), 81-88.

Stuebe, A. M., Rich-Edwards, J. W., Willett, W. C., Manson, J. E., & Michels, K. B. (2005). Duration of lactation and incidence of type 2 diabetes. *Journal of the American Medical Association, 294*(20), 2601-2610.

Stuebe, A. M., & Schwarz, E. B. (2010). The risks and benefits of infant feeding practices for women and their children. *Journal of Perinatology, 30*(3), 155-162.

Takci, S., Gulmez, D., Yigit, S., Dogan, O., & Hascelik, G. (2013). Container type and bactericidal activity of human milk during refrigerated storage. *Journal of Human Lactation, 29*(3), 406-411.

Walker, M. (2011). *Breastfeeding and employment.* Amarillo, TX: Hale Publishing.

Walsh, W. (2011). *Single babe breastfeeding: It CAN be done!* Retrieved from: http://www.bestforbabes.org/single-babe-breast feeding-it-can-be-done

Wang, W., Parker, K., & Taylor, P. (2013). *Breadwinner moms.* Washington, DC: Pew Research Center.

West, D., & Marasco, L. (2009). *The breastfeeding mother's guide to making more milk.* New York: McGraw Hill.

Williamson, M. T., & Murti, P. K. (1996). Effects of storage, time, temperature, and composition of containers on biologic components of human milk. *Journal of Human Lactation, 12*(1), 31-35.

Wilson-Clay, B., & Hoover, K. (2008). *The breastfeeding atlas* (4th Ed.). Manchaca, TX: LactNews Press.

World Health Organization. (WHO). (2010). *Infant and young child feeding.* Retrieved from: http://www.who.int/mediacen tre/factsheets/fs342/en/index.html

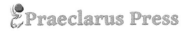
Praeclarus Press

Working and Breastfeeding Made Simple

Nancy Mohrbacher, IBCLC, FILCA

With its evidence-based insights, *Working and Breastfeeding Made Simple* takes the mystery out of pumping and milk production. Written by an international breastfeeding expert, it puts you in control of your own experience with straightforward explanations of how milk is made and what you can do to reach your own best level.

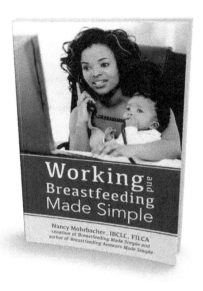

Whether your maternity leave is long, short, or in between, it includes what you need to know every step of the way. New concepts such as "The Magic Number" explain how to tailor your daily routine to your body's response. It also includes pumping strategies that can increase your milk yields by nearly 50%.

To order a copy, access http://goo.gl/Kgv6EX, or scan the QR code below.

Tips from employed mothers provide the wisdom of hindsight. No matter what your work setting or whether you stay close to home or travel regularly, this book provides the essentials you need to reach your personal breastfeeding goals.